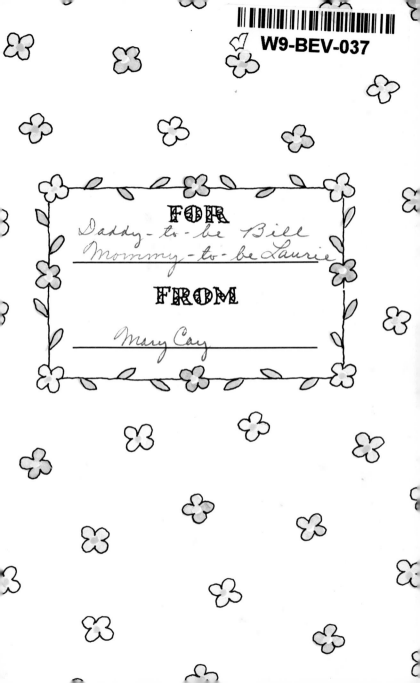

W9-BEV-037

FOR

Daddy-to-be Bill
Mommy-to-be Laurie

FROM

Mary Cay

EXPECTING

Written and Illustrated by
Dolli Tingle

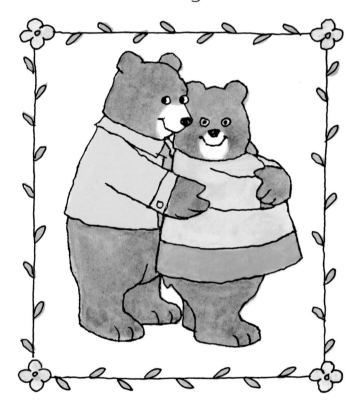

Our record of what happened
While we waited for baby

The C.R. Gibson Company, Norwalk, Connecticut 06856

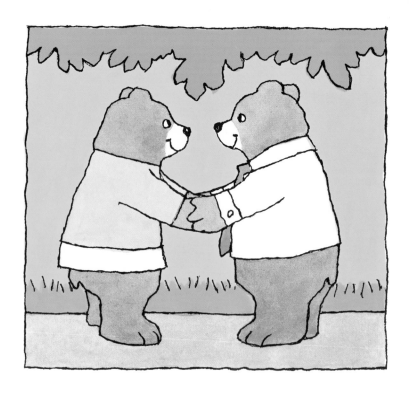

What wonderful news we have had today.
Our own little baby is on the way.

It's a thrill and a joy to know that we
Are really becoming a family.

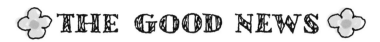

THE GOOD NEWS

When we found out:

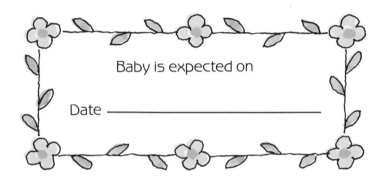

Baby is expected on

Date _____

Our reactions:

Grandparents' reactions:

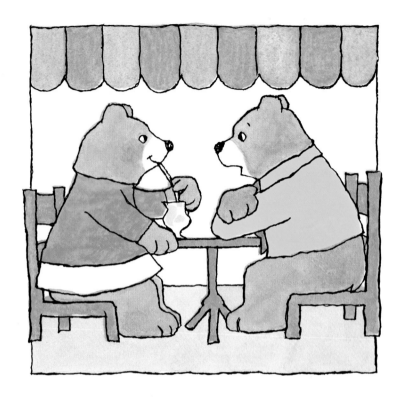

You're gaining weight.
I know you know it.
And pretty soon
You'll start to show it.
Pink ice cream sodas
Won't make a hit
When you find out
Your clothes don't fit.

DIET DO'S AND DON'TS

❀ WHAT I CRAVE ❀

I seem to remember
You being much thinner.
Perhaps you've just had
An exceptional dinner.

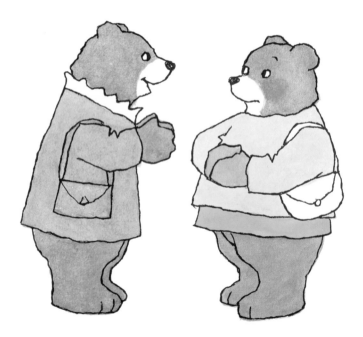

MY WEIGHT CHART

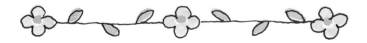

KEEPING FIT

Sit like a tailor.

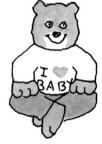

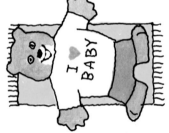

Lie on the floor. Hold your breath and stretch arms and legs. Then open mouth, slowly exhale and relax.

Lie on the floor, feet together, knees up, arms out. Roll hips to the left until knees touch the floor.

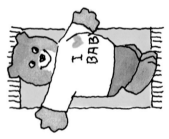

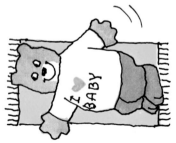

Then roll to the right in the same way. Repeat several times.

If Doctor Okays Exercises

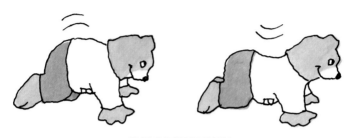

THE CAT STRETCH
On hands and knees, raise spine and back to a hump. Lower completely to a relaxed sag.

LEG LIFT
Lie on side. Lift and lower left leg. Reverse position. Lift and lower right leg.

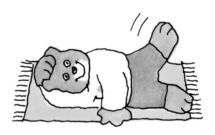

PELVIC TILT
Lie on back, arms outstretched, knees bent.

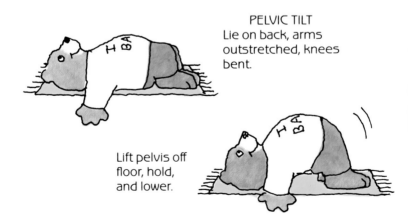

Lift pelvis off floor, hold, and lower.

MY EXERCISE PROGRAM

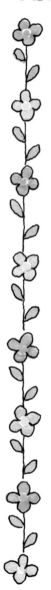

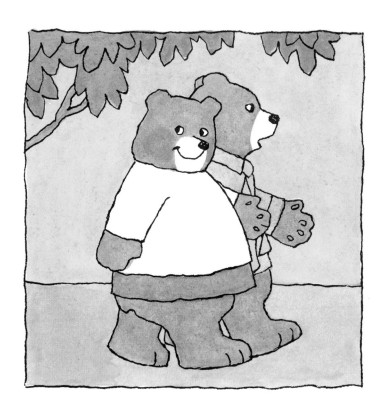

I know that you're supposed to walk.
But who said I was too?
You've got to tell our Doctor
I have other things to do!

I'm jotting down
A list of names
Like Joe and Bill
And George and James.
Or Jack or Tom
Or Bob or Earl

Or Gertrude . . .
If he is a girl.

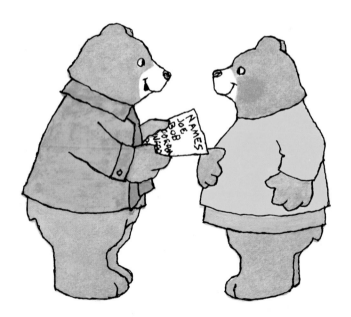

BOYS NAMES WE LIKE

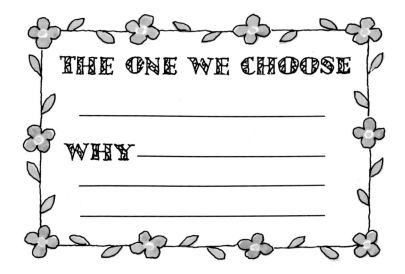

THE ONE WE CHOOSE

_____

WHY _____

_____

_____

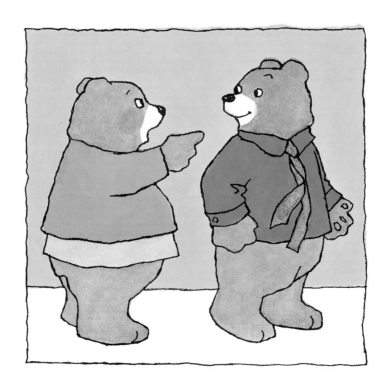

I remember you had Gertrude
Written on your list of names.
How can I be sure that Gertrude
Isn't one of your old flames?

GIRLS NAMES WE LIKE

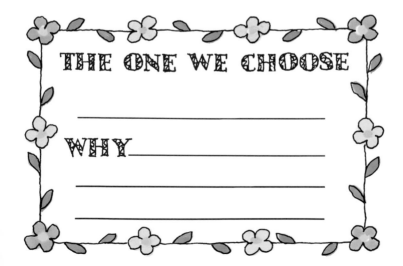

THE ONE WE CHOOSE

_____

WHY _____

_____

_____

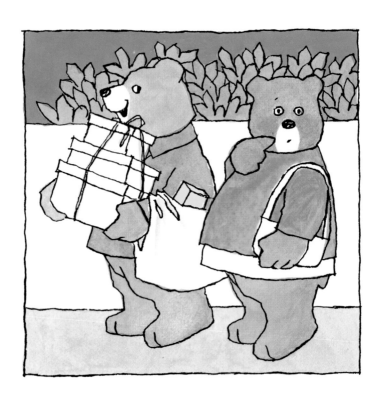

If a brand new baby
Wears a six months size
And a six months size
Is a year . . .
I'm thinkin' our baby's
Outgrown all these clothes
Even before it is here!

SHOPPING FOR BABY

- [ ] Disposable diapers
- [ ] 4-6 cotton shirts
- [ ] Stretch overalls
- [ ] Receiving blankets
- [ ] Bunting
- [ ] Booties
- [ ] 2 sweaters
- [ ] 4-6 gowns
- [ ] Diaper bag
- [ ] Baby record book

- [ ] Disposable bottles
- [ ] Baby spoon
- [ ] Bibs
- [ ] High chair

- [ ] Crib with bumpers
- [ ] Waterproof mattress
- [ ] Blankets
- [ ] Sheets

- [ ] Baby tub and changing table
- [ ] Baby towels and wash cloths
- [ ] Baby soap and shampoo
- [ ] Brush and comb
- [ ] Disposable wipes, cotton balls
- [ ] Thermometers
- [ ] Baby oil, lotion, powder
- [ ] Car seat carrier for under 3 mo.
      old baby (mandatory in some states.)

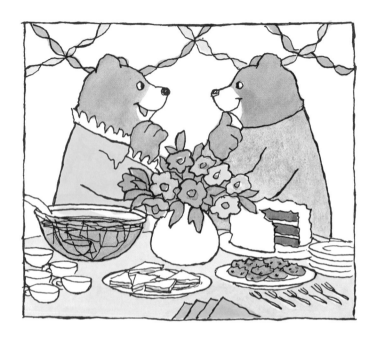

Such decorations, food and flowers!
Don't you just love baby showers?
The gift cards are so sweet and cute.
But best of all, think of the loot!

SHOWERS AND GIFTS

SHOWERS AND GIFTS

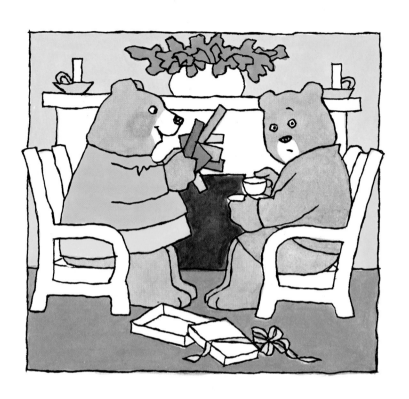

How nice of you to bring a gift
And drop in for a visit.
It must be just what baby needs.
Now tell me, dear, what is it?

You've packed all our luggage
With stuff you won't use.
We're having a baby
Not taking a cruise!

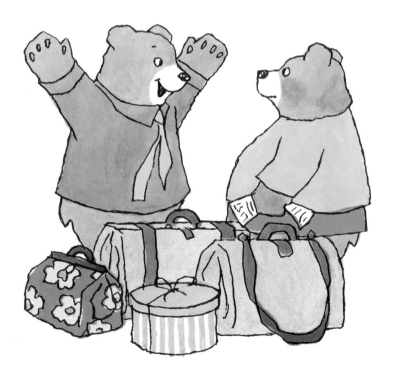

TO TAKE TO HOSPITAL

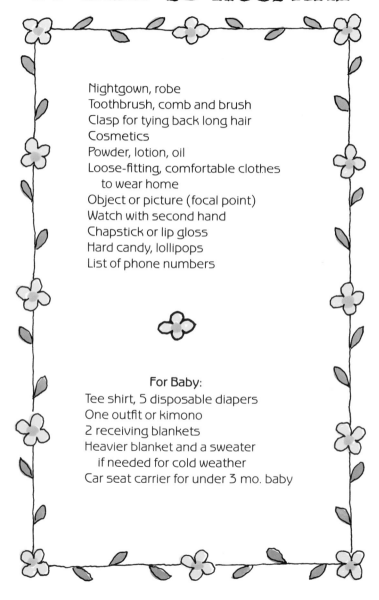

Nightgown, robe
Toothbrush, comb and brush
Clasp for tying back long hair
Cosmetics
Powder, lotion, oil
Loose-fitting, comfortable clothes
   to wear home
Object or picture (focal point)
Watch with second hand
Chapstick or lip gloss
Hard candy, lollipops
List of phone numbers

For Baby:
Tee shirt, 5 disposable diapers
One outfit or kimono
2 receiving blankets
Heavier blanket and a sweater
   if needed for cold weather
Car seat carrier for under 3 mo. baby

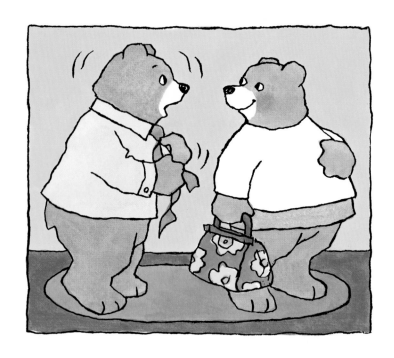

You called them up?
It's time to go?
You feel okay?
How do you know?
Don't get upset,
I'll see you through!
Now, what am I
Supposed to do?

WELCOME TO BABY!

Name _____

Born on _____

At _____ o'clock _____ M

Place _____

Weight _____ Height _____

Color of eyes _____ Hair _____

Doctor/ Nurse Midwife _____

_____

Born To:

Mother _____

Father _____

Home address _____

_____

This moment surpasses
All those we've held dear.
A wee wondrous miracle,
Baby is here!

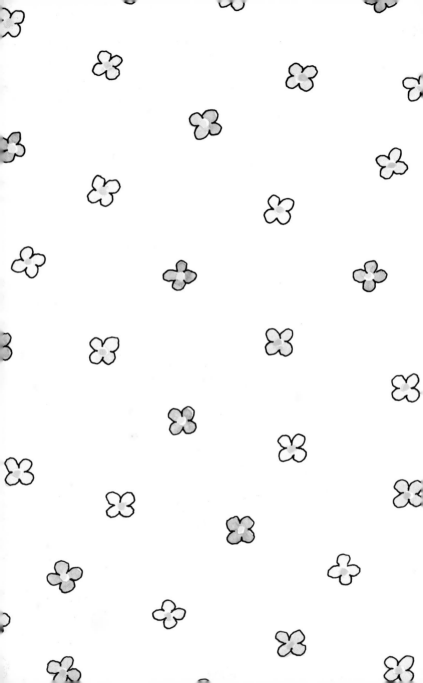